SHEET PAN COOKING COOKBOOK

To the Point 170 Pages Guideline to Become

a Sheet Pan Cooking Expert and Make

Delicious, Mouthwatering, and Hassle-Free

Meals in Less Than 30 Minutes

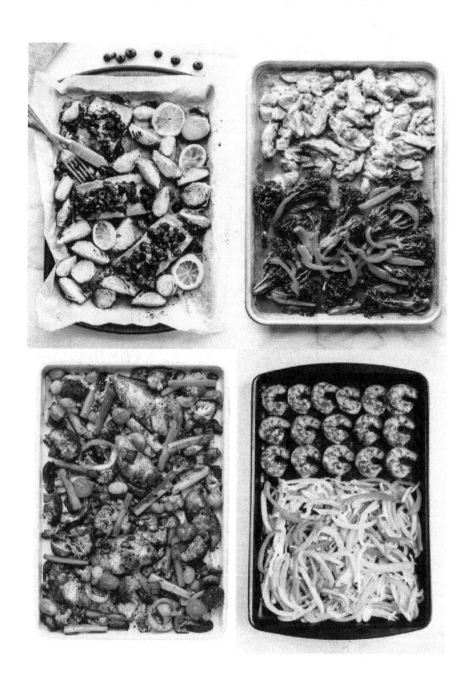

Table of Contents

INTRODUCTION

A sheet pan, preparing plate or heating sheet is a plane, rectangular metal pan utilized in an oven. It is regularly utilized for heating bread moves, cakes and level items like treats, sheet cakes, Swiss rolls and pizzas. Sheet pan cooking saves time, makes clean up less difficult, and doesn't require exorbitant stuff or extreme INGREDIENTS. Just beginning with your protein of choice, by then add vegetables, fat and flavorings, and supper at high heat until everything is splendid brown. Sheet pan dinner are brisk and easy to prepare, which suggests they can be a convenient answer for non-end of the week days when you get back home from work and have only 15 minutes to spend planning food. Not in the least like dishes masterminded in a saucepan, which require adding INGREDIENTS in a particular solicitation, irregular mixing, and changes in the temp setting, when the sheet pan is in the oven, you are free for the accompanying 15 to 60 minutes. Sheet pan dinners can be made with relatively few INGREDIENTS, normally stuff that is as of now lying around in your fridge and pantry

1. Paprika-Rubbed Sheet-Tray Chicken

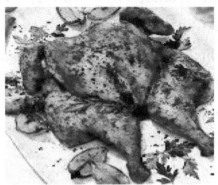

Active Time 5 Mins Total Time 1 Hour 15 Mins Yield Serves 6 (serving size: about 3 oz. chicken)

INGREDIENTS

- 1 (3 1/2- to 4-lb.) chicken, spatchcocked
- 1 tablespoon fennel seeds
- 2 teaspoons hot paprika
- 1 teaspoon kosher salt
- 1 teaspoon smoked paprika
- 1 teaspoon black pepper
- 2 garlic cloves, finely grated
- 1/4 cup olive oil
- 2 lemons, quartered

DIRECTION:

1. Preheat oven to 325°F.
2. Wipe chicken off with paper towels. Pound fennel seeds in a zest plant or with a mortar and pestle. Join fennel, hot paprika, salt,

smoked paprika, dark pepper, garlic, and olive oil in a medium bowl; rub flavor combination all over chicken. Rub any extra flavor blend onto lemon quarters.

3. Spot chicken, bosom side up, on a rimmed preparing sheet or in a 12-inch ovenproof skillet; spread lemons around chicken. Cook at 325°F for 1 hour or until chicken is delicate, lemons are delicate and jammy, and a meat thermometer embedded into thickest bit of bosom registers 160°F, treating chicken with drippings at regular intervals. Eliminate from oven; rest 15 minutes. Press lemons over chicken, or serve lemons with warm chicken.

NUTRITION FACTS

- Calories 261 Fat 14g Satfat 2g Unsatfat 11g Protein 32g Carbohydrate 1g Fiber 1g Sodium 437mg Calcium 3% DV Potassium 11% DV Sugars g Added sugars g

2. Sheet Pan Kimchi Nachos

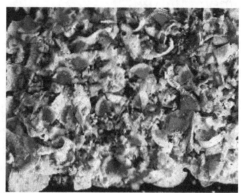

Active Time 15 Mins Total Time 20 Mins
Yield Serves 6

INGREDIENTS

- 12 ounces tortilla chips
- 2 teaspoons sesame oil
- 12 ounces ground pork
- 2 tablespoons minced shallot
- 2 cloves garlic, minced
- 1 teaspoon freshly grated ginger
- 1 1/2 teaspoons fish sauce
- 1 cup kimchi, drained and thinly sliced
- 5 tablespoons plain whole-milk Greek yogurt
- 2 teaspoons Sriracha chili sauce
- 2 teaspoons water
- 1 teaspoon seasoned rice vinegar
- 1/2 teaspoon sugar
- 1/4 teaspoon kosher salt
- 1/4 teaspoon freshly ground black pepper
- 1/2 cup thinly sliced green onion
- 1/4 cup thinly sliced watermelon radish

DIRECTION

1. Spread tortilla chips equally on a half sheet dish. Put in a safe spot.
2. Heat oil in an enormous nonstick skillet over medium. Add pork and shallot; cook 3 to 4 minutes, breaking pork into pieces with a wooden spoon. Add garlic, ginger, and fish sauce; cook 2 to 3 minutes, until pork is browned and garlic is fragrant. Utilize an opened spoon to eliminate pork from container and sprinkle equitably over chips. Spread kimchi equally over pork.
3. Consolidate Greek yogurt, Sriracha, water, vinegar, sugar, salt, and pepper in a small bowl; blend well. Spoon yogurt combination equitably over nachos. Top with green onion and watermelon radish.

NUTRITION FACTS

- Calories 410 Fat 19.5g Satfat 4.8g Monofat 3.8g Polyfat 6.7g Protein 17g Carbohydrate 44g Fiber 4g Sugars 3g Cholesterol 45mg Iron 1mg Sodium 700mg Calcium 95mg

3. Sheet Pan Baked Tilapia with Roasted Vegetables

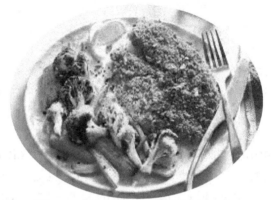

Active Time 15 Mins Total Time 30 Mins
Yield Serves 4 (serving size: 1 fillet and about 1 cup vegetables)

INGREDIENTS

- 1 tablespoon spread 1 garlic clove, minced 2 ounces entire wheat sourdough bread, finely ground 2.25 ounces all-purpose flour (around 1/2 cup) 1 egg, softly beaten 4 (6-oz.) tilapia filets 3/4 teaspoon kosher salt, isolated 1/2 teaspoon newly ground dark pepper, partitioned 1/2 tablespoons olive oil 1 (12-oz.) pkg. steam-in-sack new broccoli florets 2 medium carrots, stripped and diagonally cut Cooking splash 1 lemon, cut into wedges

DIRECTION

1. Preheat oven to 400°F.
2. Liquefy spread in a skillet over medium-high. Add garlic; cook 30 seconds. Add breadcrumbs; cook 5 minutes.

3. Spot breadcrumb combination, flour, and egg in three shallow dishes. Top fish with 1/2 teaspoon salt and 1/4 teaspoon pepper. Dig fish in flour; plunge in egg. Coat in breadcrumb combination.
4. Join staying 1/4 teaspoon salt, staying 1/4 teaspoon pepper, oil, broccoli, and carrots on a sheet dish covered with cooking shower; add fish to container. Heat at 400°F for 15 minutes or until done. Present with lemon wedges.

NUTRITION FACTS

- Calories 389 Fat 13g Satfat 4g Unsatfat 8g Protein 42g Carbohydrate 27g Fiber 5g Sugars 3g Added sugars g Sodium 598mg Calcium 11% DV Potassium 28% DV

4.   Roasted Kielbasa & Vegetables

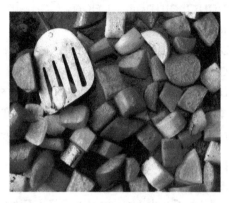

Total Time Prep: 20 min. Bake: 40 min. Makes 6 servings

INGREDIENTS

- 3 medium sweet potatoes, peeled and cut into 1-inch pieces
- 1 large sweet onion, cut into 1-inch pieces
- 4 medium carrots, cut into 1-inch pieces
- 2 tablespoons olive oil
- 1 pound smoked kielbasa or Polish sausage, halved and cut into 1-inch pieces
- 1 medium yellow summer squash, cut into 1-inch pieces
- 1 medium zucchini, cut into 1-inch pieces
- 1/4 teaspoon salt
- 1/4 teaspoon pepper

- Dijon mustard, optional

DIRECTION

1. Firstly preheat oven to 400°. Divide sweet potatoes, onion and carrots between 2 greased 15x10x1-in. baking pans. Drizzle with oil; toss to coat. Roast 25 minutes, stirring occasionally.

2. Add kielbasa, squash and zucchini to pans; sprinkle with salt and pepper. Roast until vegetables are tender, 15-20 minutes longer. Transfer to a serving bowl; toss to mix. If desired, present with mustard.

NUTRITION FACTS

- 1-2/3 cups: 378 calories, 25g fat (8g saturated fat), 51mg cholesterol, 954mg sodium, 26g carbohydrate (12g sugars, 4g fiber), 13g protein.

5. Chicken Cordon Bleu Pizza

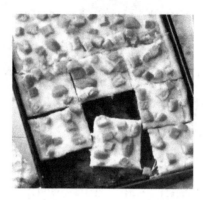

Total Time Prep/Total Time: 30 min. Makes 6

servings

INGREDIENTS

- 1 tube (13.8 ounces) refrigerated pizza crust
- 1/2 cup Alfredo sauce
- 1/4 teaspoon garlic salt
- 1 cup shredded Swiss cheese
- 1-1/2 cups cubed fully cooked ham
- 10 breaded chicken nuggets, thawed, cut into 1/2-inch pieces
- 1 cup shredded part-skim mozzarella cheese

DIRECTION

1. Preheat oven to 425°. Unroll and press dough onto bottom of a greased 15x10x1-in. pan,

pinching edges to form a rim if you want. Bake until edges are light brown, 8-10 minutes.

2. Then spread crust with Alfredo sauce; drizzle with garlic salt. Top with remaining INGREDIENTS. Bake until crust is golden brown and cheese is melted, 8-10 minutes.

NUTRITION FACTS

- 1 serving: 438 calories, 20g fat (9g saturated fat), 65mg cholesterol, 1386mg sodium, 39g carbohydrate (5g sugars, 2g fiber), 27g protein.

6.   Double Nut Baklava

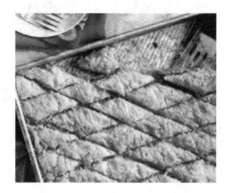

Total Time Prep: 25 min. Bake: 30 min. + standing
Makes About 3 dozen

INGREDIENTS

- 1-1/4 cups improved shredded coconut, toasted
- 1/2 cup finely chopped macadamia nuts
- 1/2 cup finely chopped walnuts
- 1/2 cup pressed brown sugar
- 1 teaspoon ground allspice
- 1-1/4 cups margarine, dissolved
- 1 bundle phyllo batter (16 ounces, 14x9-inch-sheet size), defrosted
- 1 cup sugar
- 1/2 cup water
- 1/4 cup nectar

DIRECTION

1. In a huge bowl, join the initial five INGREDIENTS; put in a safe spot. Brush a 13x9-in. heating skillet with a portion of the margarine. Unroll the sheets of phyllo batter; trim to find a way into skillet.
2. Layer 10 sheets of phyllo in arranged container, brushing each with margarine.

(Continue to remain batter covered with saran wrap and a moist towel to keep it from drying out.) Sprinkle with 33% of the nut combination. Rehash layers twice. Top with five phyllo sheets, brushing each with spread. Brush top sheet of phyllo with margarine.

3. Using a sharp blade, cut into jewel shapes. Prepare at 350° for 30-35 minutes or until brilliant brown. Cool totally on a wire rack.
4. In a little pot, bring the sugar, water and nectar to a bubble. Diminish heat; stew for 5 minutes. Pour hot syrup over baklava. Cover and let stand for the time being.

NUTRITION FACTS
- 1 piece: 174 calories, 10g fat (5g saturated fat), 17mg cholesterol, 134mg sodium, 20g carbohydrate (12g sugars, 1g fiber), 2g protein.

7. Tomato-Onion Phyllo Pizza

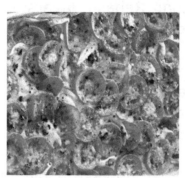

Total Time Prep: 20 min. Bake: 20 min. Makes 28 slices

INGREDIENTS
- 5 tablespoons margarine, softened
- 14 sheets phyllo mixture (14x9 in.)
- 7 tablespoons ground Parmesan cheddar, isolated
- 1 cup shredded part-skim mozzarella cheddar
- 1 cup meagerly cut onion
- 1 pound plum tomatoes, cut
- 1-1/2 teaspoons minced new oregano or 1/2 teaspoon dried oregano
- 1 teaspoon minced new thyme or 1/4 teaspoon dried thyme
- Salt and pepper to taste

DIRECTION
1. Preheat oven to 375°. Brush a 15x10x1-in. heating skillet with a portion of the softened spread. Unroll phyllo batter; cut stack into a 10-1/2x9-in. square shape. Dispose of scraps.
2. Line base and sides of arranged skillet with 2 sheets of phyllo mixture (sheets will cover

marginally). Brush with margarine and sprinkle with 1 tablespoon Parmesan cheddar. Rehash layers multiple times. (Keep batter covered with a moist towel until prepared to use to keep it from drying out.)

3. Top with layers of residual phyllo batter; brush with outstanding spread. Sprinkle with mozzarella cheddar; mastermind onion and tomatoes over cheddar. Sprinkle with oregano, thyme, salt, pepper and remaining Parmesan cheddar. Heat until edges are brilliant brown, 20-25 minutes.

NUTRITION FACTS

- 1 slice: 54 calories, 3g fat (2g saturated fat), 9mg cholesterol, 87mg sodium, 4g carbohydrate (1g sugars, 0 fiber), 2g protein.

8. Ragin' Cajun Eggplant and Shrimp Skillet

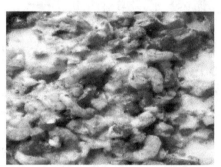

Total Time Prep: 30 min. Bake: 35 min. Makes 4 servings

INGREDIENTS

- 1 medium eggplant, stripped and cut into 1/2-inch blocks
- 3 tablespoons olive oil
- 2 celery ribs, diced
- 1 medium onion, diced
- 1 little green pepper, cultivated and diced
- 3 plum tomatoes, diced
- 1 teaspoon squashed red pepper chips
- 1/2 teaspoon pepper
- 12 ounces uncooked shell-on shrimp (31-40 for every pound), stripped and deveined
- 1/2 cup prepared bread scraps
- 1-1/2 cups shredded part-skim mozzarella cheddar

DIRECTION

1. Spot eggplant in an enormous pan; add water to cover. Heat to the point of boiling. Diminish heat; stew, covered, until delicate, 3-4 minutes. Channel.

2. Preheat oven to 350°. In an ovenproof skillet, heat oil over medium-high heat. Add celery, onion and green pepper; saute until delicate, around 5 minutes. Diminish heat to medium; mix in tomatoes and eggplant. Saute 5 minutes. Mix in flavors. Add shrimp and bread morsels; saute 5 minutes longer, mixing great.
3. Prepare 30 minutes. Eliminate skillet from oven; top with cheddar. Prepare 5 minutes more.

NUTRITION FACTS

- 1 serving: 399 calories, 21g fat (7g saturated fat), 131mg cholesterol, 641mg sodium, 26g carbohydrate (9g sugars, 5g fiber), 28g protein.

9. Spicy Roasted Sausage, Potatoes and Peppers

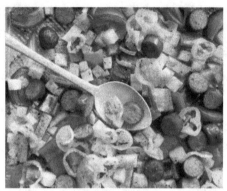

Total Time Prep: 20 min. Bake: 30 min. Makes 4 servings

INGREDIENTS

- 1 pound potatoes (about 2 medium), peeled and cut into 1/2-inch cubes
- 1 package (12 ounces) fully cooked andouille chicken sausage links or flavor of your choice, cut into 1-inch pieces
- 1 medium red onion, cut into wedges
- 1 medium sweet red pepper, cut into 1-inch pieces
- 1 medium green pepper, cut into 1-inch pieces
- 1/2 cup pickled pepper rings
- 1 tablespoon olive oil
- 1/2 to 1 teaspoon Creole seasoning
- 1/4 teaspoon pepper

DIRECTION

1. Firstly preheat oven to 400°. In a large bowl, combine potatoes, sausage, onion, red pepper, green pepper and pepper rings. Combine oil,

Creole seasoning and pepper; sprinkle over potato mixture and toss to coat.
2. Transfer to a 15x10x1-in. baking pan coated with cooking spray. Roast until vegetables are tender, stirring occasionally, 30-35 minutes.

NUTRITION FACTS
- 1-1/2 cups: 257 calories, 11g fat (3g saturated fat), 65mg cholesterol, 759mg sodium, 24g carbohydrate (5g sugars, 3g fiber), 17g protein. Diabetic Exchanges: 3 lean meat, 1 starch, 1 vegetable, 1 fat.

10. Sausage Stuffing

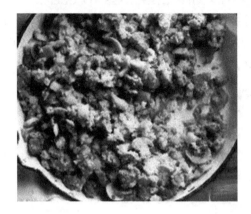

Total Time Prep/Total Time: 25 min. Makes 8 servings

INGREDIENTS
- 1 pound mass pork sausage
- 1-1/4 cups chopped celery
- 1/2 cup chopped onion
- 1/2 cup cut new mushrooms
- 1 enormous garlic clove, minced
- 1-1/2 cups diminished sodium chicken stock
- 1 teaspoon scoured sage
- 1 bundle (6 ounces) stuffing blend

DIRECTION
1. In an enormous skillet, cook the frankfurter, celery, onion and mushrooms over medium heat until meat is not, at this point pink. Add garlic; cook brief longer; channel. Mix in stock and sage.
2. Heat to the point of boiling. Mix in stuffing blend. Cover and eliminate from the heat; let represent 5 minutes. Cushion with a fork.

3. Dried spices have their place in a lot of recipes, however stuffing isn't one of them. Attempt a blend of new parsley, sage, rosemary and thyme,
4. Custom made bread garnishes will truly make your stuffing sparkle. Any portion of bread will work, top choices are nation portion, sourdough, brioche or rye portion. Cut the bread into 1-inch solid shapes and throw them into a 300°F oven until they're dry and fresh, around 45 minutes. Get more tips for best-truly stuffing.

NUTRITION FACTS

- 1 serving: 219 calories, 13g fat (4g saturated fat), 21mg cholesterol, 756mg sodium, 18g carbohydrate (4g sugars, 1g fiber), 7g protein.

11. Sheet pan Parmesan Chicken

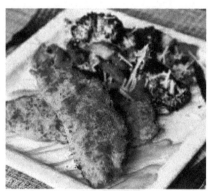

Total Time Prep: 20 min. Bake: 20 min. Makes 4 servings

INGREDIENTS

- 4 boneless skinless chicken bosom parts (6 ounces each)
- 3 teaspoons olive oil, separated
- 1 teaspoon dried rosemary, squashed
- 1/2 teaspoon dried thyme
- 1/2 teaspoon pepper
- 2 jars (14 ounces each) water-stuffed artichoke hearts, depleted and quartered
- 1 medium onion, coarsely chopped
- 1/2 cup white wine or decreased sodium chicken stock
- 2 garlic cloves, chopped
- 1/4 cup shredded Parmesan cheddar
- 1 lemon, cut into 8 cuts
- 2 green onions, daintily cut

DIRECTION

1. Preheat oven to 375°. Spot chicken in a 15x10x1-in. preparing dish covered with

cooking shower; sprinkle with 1-1/2 teaspoons oil. In a small bowl, blend rosemary, thyme and pepper; sprinkle half over chicken.

2. In a huge bowl, consolidate artichoke hearts, onion, wine, garlic, remaining oil and remaining spice blend; throw to cover. Orchestrate around chicken. Sprinkle chicken with cheddar; top with lemon cuts.

3. Broil until a thermometer embedded in chicken peruses 165°, 20-25 minutes. Sprinkle with green onions.

NUTRITION FACTS

- 1 chicken breast half with 3/4 cup artichoke mixture: 339 calories, 9g fat (3g saturated fat), 98mg cholesterol, 667mg sodium, 18g carbohydrate (2g sugars, 1g fiber), 42g protein. Diabetic Exchanges: 5 lean meat, 1 vegetable, 1 fat, 1/2 starch

12. Sheet Pan Honey-Soy Salmon Dinner

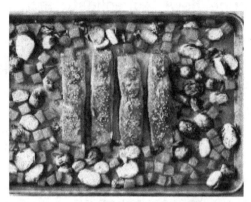

Active Time 15 Mins Total Time 42 Mins Yield Serves 4 (1 salmon fillet, about 2/3 cup squash, and 2/3 cup Brussels sprouts)

INGREDIENTS

- Cooking splash 1/2 tablespoon lower-sodium soy sauce or tamari 3 tablespoons olive oil, separated 1 tablespoon nectar 1 tablespoon new lime juice (from 1 lime) 2 cloves garlic, minced, partitioned 1/2 teaspoon newly ground ginger 4 (5 oz) skin-on salmon filets 2 1/2 cups butternut squash, stripped and cubed 12 ounces Brussels grows, managed and split 1/2 teaspoon legitimate salt 1/2 teaspoon newly ground dark pepper 1/4 teaspoon smoked paprika 1 tablespoon cut green onion 1 teaspoon
sesame seeds

DIRECTION

1. Stage 1
2. Preheat oven to 400°F. Coat a 13 x 18-inch half sheet dish with cooking splash.

3. Stage 2
4. Consolidate soy sauce, 1 tablespoon of the oil, nectar, lime juice, 1 clove of garlic, and ginger in an enormous bowl. Spot salmon in bowl. Throw to cover. Put in a safe spot.
5. Stage 3
6. In a different bowl, consolidate remaining 2 tablespoons of oil, remaining clove of garlic, butternut squash, Brussels sprouts, salt, pepper, and paprika. Throw to cover. Spread on preparing sheet, abstaining from congestion. Heat at 400°F for 12 minutes. Mix vegetables and push to edges of skillet, making an open place.
7. Stage 4
8. Spot marinated salmon filets in the open community space of container. Pour any extra marinade over salmon. Prepare at 400° for 15 minutes. Top salmon with green onion and sesame seeds. Present with squash and Brussels sprouts.

NUTRITION FACTS
- Calories 392 Fat 19.5g Satfat 2.9g Monofat 10.4g Polyfat 4.8g Protein 33g Carbohydrate 23g Fiber 5g Sugars 8g Cholesterol 78mg Iron 3mg Sodium 641mg Calcium 99mg

13. SHEET PAN TERIYAKI SALMON AND VEGETABLES

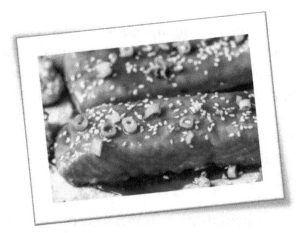

PREP TIME:15 mins COOK TIME: 20 mins TOTAL TIME: 35 mins

INGREDIENTS

- For vegetables:
- 2 cups reduced down broccoli florets
- 10 scaled down sweet rainbow peppers, cultivated and divided
- 1 tablespoon sesame oil
- ¼ teaspoon genuine salt
- Newly ground dark pepper, to taste
- For salmon:
- 2 (4-ounce) wild salmon filets
- 1 teaspoon sesame oil
- 1 garlic clove, ground
- ½ teaspoon ground ginger
- 2 tablespoons diminished sodium soy sauce, or sans gluten soy sauce
- 1 teaspoon unseasoned rice vinegar

- 1 teaspoon brown sugar
- For decorate:
- ½ teaspoon toasted sesame seeds
- 1 enormous scallion, chopped

DIRECTION

1. Preheat oven to 400F degrees. Cover an enormous sheet skillet with foil or material, gently shower olive oil and put in a safe spot.
2. In the mean time, join sesame oil, garlic, ginger, soy sauce, vinegar and brown sugar in a little bowl and blend. Fill a huge ziplock sack and add salmon, marinate 10 minutes.
3. salmon in marinade
4. In a medium bowl, throw broccoli and peppers with 1 tablespoon sesame oil, ¼ teaspoon salt and pepper. Spread them uniformly on arranged sheet container and meal for 10 minutes.
5. Eliminate veggies from oven, throw, and move them over somewhat to account for the salmon. Spot the salmon on the sheet skillet, holding the marinade and get back to oven, broil an extra 7 to 8 minutes, or until salmon is simply cooked through.
6. While salmon is cooking, heat a little skillet over low heat. Pour the leftover marinade and stew mixing until the sauce has thickened somewhat, around 1 to 1/2 minutes.
7. Brush sauce over salmon and sprinkle filets with sesame seeds and scallions. Present with veggies as an afterthought.

NUTRITION FACTS

- Serving: 1filet with 1 cup veggies, Calories: 326kcal, Carbohydrates: 17g, Protein: 27g, Fat: 17g, Saturated Fat: 2.5g, Cholesterol: 62mg, Sodium: 758mg, Fiber: 4g, Sugar: 4gBlue Smart Points:4Green Smart Points:7Purple Smart Points:4Points +:8

14. Crispy Sheet Pan Salmon with Lemony Asparagus and Carrots

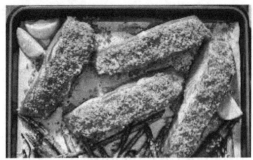

Active:20 mins Total:40 mins Yield: Serves 4 (serving size: 1 fillet, about 4 oz. vegetables)

INGREDIENTS

- 4 (6-oz.) skin-on salmon filets
- ¼ cup mayonnaise
- 2 tablespoons Dijon mustard
- 1 tablespoon chopped new dill
- 1 ½ teaspoons lemon zing (from 1 lemon), partitioned
- ¾ teaspoon genuine salt, separated
- ¾ teaspoon dark pepper, partitioned
- ¼ cup panko (Japanese-style breadcrumbs)
- Cooking splash
- ½ pound new asparagus, managed and split transversely
- 1 (8-oz.) pkg. little carrots with tops, cut longwise
- 2 tablespoons unsalted margarine, liquefied
- Lemon wedges

DIRECTION

Stage 1

1. Preheat oven to 425°F. Line a rimmed preparing sheet with material paper. Spot salmon, skin side down, on portion of arranged preparing sheet. Mix together mayonnaise, mustard, dill, 1 teaspoon of the lemon zing, 1/4 teaspoon of the salt, and 1/4 teaspoon of the pepper in a medium bowl. Spread over salmon filets in an even layer; top with panko, and press gently to follow. Splash with cooking shower.

2. Stage 2

3. Throw together asparagus, carrots, margarine, and staying 1/2 teaspoon every one of lemon zing, salt, and pepper in a medium bowl. Spot vegetables on void side of preparing sheet. Heat in preheated oven until salmon is cooked through and vegetables are delicate, around 18 minutes. Present with lemon wedges.

NUTRITION FACTS

- 1 serving: 219 calories, 13g fat (4g saturated fat), 21mg cholesterol, 756mg sodium, 18g carbohydrate (4g sugars, 1g fiber), 7g protein.

15. Sheet pan Asian chicken

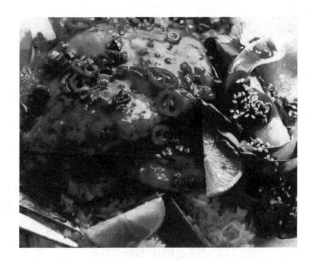

Prep: 5 mins Cook: 8 mins , serving: 8

INGREDIENTS

- CHICKEN:
- 500g/1lb breast filets, skinless and boneless (2 huge) (Note 1 different cuts)
- 1/2 tsp each salt and pepper
- 1 1/2 tbsp rice flour, or universally handy/plain flour (Note 2)
- 1 1/2 tbsp oil , vegetable or canola
- SAUCE:
- 2 tsp sesame oil
- 2 garlic cloves , finely minced
- 2 tsp ginger , finely minced
- 1 tsp bean stew chips/red pepper pieces (decrease for less fiery)
- 1/2 cup water

- 3 tbsp sriracha (sub ketchup for not fiery, Note 3)
- 1 tbsp soy sauce , light or universally handy (Note 4)
- 1/4 cup nectar (sub brown sugar)
- 3 tbsp lime juice (sub 2 tbsp rice vinegar)
- Enhancements (CHOOSE):
- Green onion (finely cut), sesame seeds, new stew, lime wedges

DIRECTION
1. CHICKEN:
2. Season: Cut every chicken bosom fifty-fifty on a level plane to frame 4 steaks absolute. Sprinkle each side with salt, pepper and rice flour, shaking off overabundance.
3. Sear: Heat oil in a huge skillet over high heat. Add chicken and cook for 2 minutes. Turn and cook the opposite side for 2 minutes, at that point eliminate to a plate.
4. Tacky Chili SAUCE:
5. Sesame oil: Allow the skillet to cool somewhat then re-visitation of the oven on medium. Add sesame oil and heat.
6. Garlic and ginger: Add garlic and ginger, cook for 15 seconds.
7. Bean stew chips: Add stew pieces and cook for 30 seconds until garlic is brilliant.
8. Sriracha, soy and nectar: Turn heat up to medium-high. Add water, sriracha, soy sauce and nectar, mix well, scratching the base of the dish to break down every one of the brilliant pieces into the fluid.

9. Stew for 2 minutes until it decrease to a thick syrup. Add lime juice, at that point stew for a further 30 seconds until it thickens back to a thick syrup.
10. Coat chicken: Turn heat off. Return chicken to dish, going to cover in sauce.
11. Serve chicken, finishing off with residual sauce in skillet, embellished with green onions, sesame seed and additional lime wedges, whenever wanted.
12. Formula Notes:
13. Chicken – Boneless and skinless thighs and tenderloins additionally work, utilize 500g/1lb. Try not to slice down the middle, utilize entire pieces.
14. Thighs will take more time to cook through, around 4 minutes on the primary side, 3 minutes on the subsequent side;
15. Tenderloins are (commonly) more modest so they should take the around a similar time as bosom.
16. Inside temperature of cooked chicken:
17. Bosom and tenderloin: 65°C/150°F
18. Thigh: 75°C/167°F
19. Rice flour – Yields a decent, firm outside layer onto which the tacky stew sauce sticks. Without it, the sauce simply sneaks off the chicken. It is anything but a serious deal in the event that you don't have it – sub plain/generally useful flour. Rice flour is simply somewhat crisper. ☺
20. Sriracha – This adds fieriness just as different flavors like vinegar and garlic into the sauce, in addition to it thickens the sauce.

21. On the off chance that you need less zesty, sub some of it with ketchup. In the event that you sub every last bit of it, the dish turns out to be very sweet so add a scramble of additional lime to redress (it's likewise absolutely not what this formula is proposed to be, but rather it's as yet delicious!)

22. In the event that you need fiery however don't have sriracha, additionally sub with ketchup in addition to some other hot sauce to taste, or cayenne pepper or more stew chips.

23. Soy sauce – Use universally handy or light, don't utilize dim soy sauce (shading and flavor excessively extraordinary). More on various soy sauces here.

24. Capacity – Lean meats like bosom and tenderloin are in every case best served newly made. However, it will save for 3 – 4 days in the cooler. Best to reheat in the microwave, and delicately, so you don't overcook it!

NUTRITION FACTS

- Calories: 287cal (14%)Carbohydrates: 21g (7%)Protein: 27g (54%)Fat: 11g (17%)Saturated   Fat: 1g (6%)Trans Fat: 1gCholesterol: 80mg (27%)Sodium: 948 mg (41%)Potassium: 522mg (15%)Fiber: 1g (4%)Sugar: 18g (20%)Vitamin A: 59IU (1%)Vitamin C: 13mg (16%)Calcium: 15mg (2%)Iron: 1mg (6%)

16. Whole Roasted Red Snapper with Potatoes and Onions

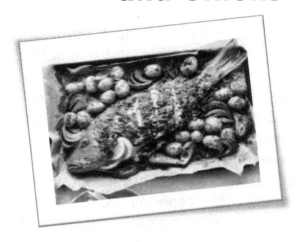

Active:25 mins Total:55 mins Yield: Serves 4 (serving size: about 4 oz. fish, 2 potatoes, 2 red onion wedges)

INGREDIENTS
- 1 ½ cups approximately pressed new level leaf parsley leaves
- 1 medium shallot (around 2 oz.), generally chopped
- 3 garlic cloves, generally chopped
- 1 tablespoon new thyme leaves
- 1 ½ teaspoons lemon zing (from 1 lemon)
- ½ teaspoon squashed red pepper
- ¾ cup olive oil
- 2 ¾ teaspoons legitimate salt, separated
- 1 pound child gold potatoes (around 8 potatoes)
- 1 little red onion (around 8 oz.), cut the long way into 1-in. wedges

- 1 (3-lb.) entire red snapper, cleaned, scaled, gutted, and blades managed
- Lemon wedges, for serving

DIRECTION
1. Stage 1
2. Preheat oven to 425°F. Line a rimmed heating sheet with material paper. Put in a safe spot.
3. Stage 2
4. Cycle parsley, shallot, garlic, thyme, lemon zing, and red pepper in a food processor until finely chopped, around 15 seconds. Add oil, and interaction until very much fused, around 15 seconds. Throw together potatoes, onion wedges, 2 tablespoons of the parsley combination, and 1 teaspoon of the salt in an enormous bowl.
5. Stage 3
6. Cut 3 (2-inch-long) cuts askew on the two sides of fish, slicing right deep down on the two sides. Rub outside and within cuts with 1 cup of the parsley blend and staying 1 3/4 teaspoons salt; place fish on arranged heating sheet. Spread potato blend around fish. Prepare in preheated oven until fish is murky and flaky and vegetables are delicate, around 30 minutes.
7. Stage 4
8. Shower fish with remaining 1/4 cup parsley combination. Present with lemon wedges.

NUTRITION FACTS
- 1 serving: 624 calories, 32g fat (10g saturated fat), 136mg cholesterol, 742mg sodium, 39g

carbohydrate (1g sugars, 6g fiber), 44g protein.

17. "Fried" Chicken with Broccoli and Sweet Potato Wedges

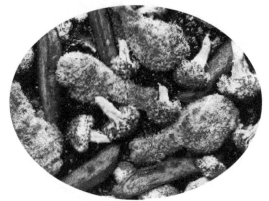

Prep time : 30 min Serves 4

INGREDIENTS

- 8 (3 1/2-oz.) chicken drumsticks, cleaned 1 tablespoon new lemon juice 1/8 teaspoons kosher salt, isolated 1/2 teaspoon poultry preparing 1 teaspoon garlic powder, separated 1/8 teaspoon newly ground dark pepper 2 huge eggs, gently thumped 1 cup panko (Japanese breadcrumbs) 1/2 ounces Parmesan cheddar, ground (around 1/3 cup) 1 teaspoon dried oregano 1 teaspoon dried parsley pieces (optional) Cooking splash 2 (7-oz.) yams, each cut into 8 wedges 2 tablespoons olive oil, partitioned 1/2 teaspoon paprika 1/2 teaspoon bean stew powder 7 cups broccoli florets (around 12 oz.) 1 garlic clove, squashed or ground 5 lemon wedges

DIRECTION:

1. Preheat oven to 425°F.

2. Spot chicken in an enormous bowl. Shower with lemon squeeze, and sprinkle with 3/8 teaspoon salt, poultry preparing, 1/2 teaspoon garlic powder, and dark pepper; throw to join.
3. Spot eggs in a shallow dish. Consolidate panko, Parmesan, oregano, and parsley, if using, in another shallow dish. Plunge every drumstick in eggs at that point dig in panko blend. Spot drumsticks on a rimmed heating sheet covered with cooking shower; dispose of outstanding egg and panko blend. Coat highest points of drumsticks with cooking splash. Prepare at 425°F for 15 minutes.
4. Consolidate potatoes, 1 tablespoon oil, staying 1/2 teaspoon garlic powder, paprika, bean stew powder, and 3/8 teaspoon salt; throw to cover. Mastermind potatoes on one portion of another rimmed preparing sheet covered with cooking shower. Spot in oven with chicken, and heat at 425°F for 10 minutes.
5. Consolidate broccoli, staying 1 tablespoon oil, garlic clove, and staying 3/8 teaspoon salt. Eliminate heating sheet with potatoes from oven; turn potatoes over, and add broccoli to other portion of container. Spot in oven with chicken, and heat at 425°F for 20 minutes or until chicken and potatoes are finished. Crush 1 lemon wedge over broccoli. Serve remaining lemon wedges with the dinner.

NUTRITION FACTS
- Calories 425 Fat 17g Sat fat 4g Unsatfat 12g Protein 34g Carbohydrate 35g Fiber 7g Sodium

902mg Calcium 19% DV Potassium 31% DV Sugars 7g Added sugars 9g

18. Honey-Soy-Glazed Salmon with Veggies and Oranges

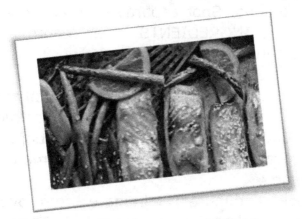

Hands-On:25 mins Total:25 mins Yield:Makes 4 servings

INGREDIENTS

- 4 tablespoons nectar
- 1 tablespoon soy sauce
- 1 tablespoon Dijon mustard
- 1 teaspoon prepared rice wine vinegar
- ¼ teaspoon dried squashed red pepper
- 1 pound new medium asparagus
- 8 ounces new green beans, managed
- 1 little orange, cut into 1/4-to 1/2-inch cuts
- 1 tablespoon olive oil
- 1 teaspoon legitimate salt
- ¼ teaspoon newly ground dark pepper
- 4 (5-to 6-oz.) new salmon filets
- Topping: toasted sesame seeds

DIRECTION

1. Stage 1

2. Preheat oven with oven rack 6 crawls from heat. Whisk together nectar and next 4 INGREDIENTS in a little bowl.
3. Stage 2
4. Snap off and dispose of intense closures of asparagus. Spot asparagus, green beans, and next 4 INGREDIENTS in an enormous bowl, and throw to cover.
5. Stage 3
6. Spot salmon in focus of a substantial aluminum foil-lined sheet container. Brush salmon with around 2 Tbsp. nectar combination. Spread asparagus combination around salmon.
7. Stage 4
8. Cook 4 minutes; eliminate from oven, and brush salmon with around 2 Tbsp. nectar combination. Get back to oven, and sear 4 minutes more. Eliminate from oven, and brush salmon with remaining nectar blend. Get back to oven, and cook 2 minutes more. Serve right away.

NUTRITION FACTS

- 359 calories, 8g fat (4g saturated fat), 56mg cholesterol, 372mg sodium, 45g carbohydrate (19g sugars, 6g fiber), 31g protein. Diabetic Exchanges: 3 starch, 3 lean meat, 1 fat.

19. Sheet Pan Hawaiian Shrimp

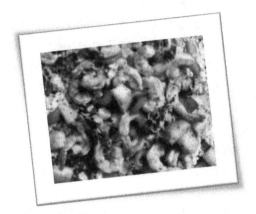

Active:15 mins Total:20 mins Yield:Serves 4 (serving size: about 5 shrimp and 1 cup rice mixture)

INGREDIENTS

- 2 (8.8-oz.) pkg. precooked jasmine rice
- 3 tablespoons canola oil
- 2 cups fresh pineapple chunks (about 8 oz.)
- 1 large red bell pepper, cut into 1-in. pieces
- 1 ¼ pounds raw large shrimp, peeled and deveined
- 3 tablespoons lower-sodium soy sauce
- 2 tablespoons light brown sugar
- 1 ½ tablespoons unseasoned rice vinegar
- ½ teaspoon black pepper
- ½ cup loosely packed fresh cilantro leaves

DIRECTION

1. Step 1
2. Preheat oven to 450°F. Place a rimmed baking sheet in oven (do not remove pan while oven preheats).
3. Step 2

4. Place rice and oil in a bowl. Using your fingers, break apart rice and coat with oil. Carefully remove pan from oven; spread rice mixture in an even layer in center of pan. Bake in preheated oven for 5 minutes; stir. Top rice with pineapple and bell pepper; bake at 450°F for 5 minutes. Arrange shrimp over rice mixture; bake at 450°F until shrimp are done, about 6 minutes.
5. Step 3
6. Place soy sauce, sugar, and vinegar in a microwave-safe bowl. Microwave at high 45 seconds. Whisk until sugar dissolves. Drizzle over pan. Add black pepper; toss. Sprinkle with cilantro.

NUTRITION FACTS

- Per Serving: 505 calories; fat 14g; saturated fat 1g; protein 26g; carbohydrates 68g; fiber 2g; sugars 13g; added sugar 7g; sodium 655mg.

20. Sheet pan Salmon Veggie Packets

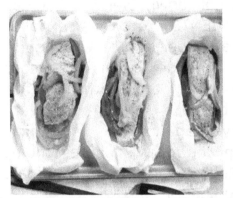

Total Time Prep/Total Time: 30 min.Makes 4 servings

INGREDIENTS

- 2 tablespoons white wine
- 1 tablespoon olive oil
- 1/4 teaspoon salt
- 1/4 teaspoon pepper
- 2 medium sweet yellow peppers, julienned
- 2 cups new sugar snap peas, managed
- SALMON:
- 2 tablespoons white wine
- 1 tablespoon olive oil
- 1 tablespoon ground lemon zing
- 1/2 teaspoon salt
- 1/4 teaspoon pepper
- 4 salmon filets (6 ounces each)
- 1 medium lemon, split

DIRECTION

1. Preheat oven to 400°. Cut four 18x15-in. bits of material paper or uncompromising foil: overlay each transversely down the middle,

shaping a wrinkle. In a huge bowl, blend wine, oil, salt and pepper. Add vegetables and throw to cover.

2. In a small bowl, blend the initial five salmon INGREDIENTS. To collect, expose one piece of material paper; place a salmon filet on one side. Sprinkle with 2 teaspoons wine combination; top with one-fourth of the vegetables.

3. Overlay paper over fish and vegetables; overlap the open closures multiple times to seal. Rehash with outstanding parcels. Spot on heating sheets.

4. Heat until fish simply starts to chip effectively with a fork, 12-16 minutes, opening parcels cautiously to allow steam to get away.

5. To serve, press lemon juice over vegetables.

NUTRITION FACTS

- 1 serving: 400 calories, 23g fat (4g saturated fat), 85mg cholesterol, 535mg sodium, 13g carbohydrate (3g sugars, 3g fiber), 32g protein. Diabetic Exchanges: 5 lean meat, 1-1/2 fat, 1 vegetable.

21. Pan-Roasted Chicken and Vegetables

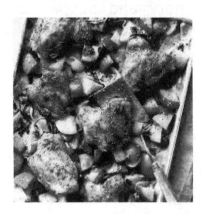

Total Time Prep: 15 min. Bake: 45 min. Makes 6 servings

INGREDIENTS

- 2 pounds red potatoes (around 6 medium), cut into 3/4-inch pieces
- 1 enormous onion, coarsely chopped
- 2 tablespoons olive oil
- 3 garlic cloves, minced
- 1-1/4 teaspoons salt, separated
- 1 teaspoon dried rosemary, squashed, isolated
- 3/4 teaspoon pepper, separated
- 1/2 teaspoon paprika
- 6 bone-in chicken thighs (around 2-1/4 pounds), skin eliminated
- 6 cups new child spinach (around 6 ounces)

DIRECTION

1. Preheat oven to 425°. In a huge bowl, consolidate potatoes, onion, oil, garlic, 3/4 teaspoon salt, 1/2 teaspoon rosemary and 1/2 teaspoon pepper; throw to cover. Move to a

15x10x1-in. preparing pan covered with cooking shower.

2. In a small bowl, blend paprika and the leftover salt, rosemary and pepper. Sprinkle chicken with paprika combination; organize over vegetables. Cook until a thermometer embedded in chicken peruses 170°-175° and vegetables are simply delicate, 35-40 minutes.

3. Eliminate chicken to a serving platter; keep warm. Top vegetables with spinach. Broil until vegetables are delicate and spinach is shriveled, 8-10 minutes longer. Mix vegetables to join; present with chicken.

4. Set up your sheet-pan supper the prior night and simply pop it into the preheated oven to prepare. This serves to profoundly enhance the chicken, a shared benefit!

5. In the event that you need a more extravagant dish, use skin-on chicken, and on the off chance that you need a lighter dish, utilize bone-in chicken breasts. Make certain to cook bone-in breasts just to 165-170 degrees, since more slender meat can get dry at higher temperatures.

NUTRITION FACTS

- 1 chicken thigh with 1 cup vegetables: 357 calories, 14g fat (3g saturated fat), 87mg cholesterol, 597mg sodium, 28g carbohydrate (3g sugars, 4g fiber), 28g protein. Diabetic Exchanges: 4 lean meat, 1-1/2 starch, 1 vegetable, 1 fat.

22. Sheet pan Pastry Chicken Bundles

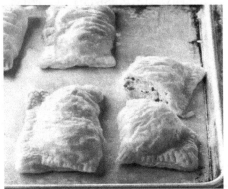

Total Time Prep: 30 min. Bake: 20 min. Makesm8 servings

INGREDIENTS

- 8 boneless skinless chicken breast halves (about 6 ounces each)
- 1 teaspoon salt
- 1/2 teaspoon pepper
- 40 large spinach leaves
- 1 carton (8 ounces) spreadable chive and onion cream cheese
- 1/2 cup chopped walnuts, toasted
- 2 sheets frozen puff pastry, thawed
- 1 large egg
- 1/2 teaspoon cold water

DIRECTION

1. Preheat oven to 400°. Cut a longwise cut in every chicken bosom half to inside 1/2 in. of the opposite side; open meat so it lies level. Cover with cling wrap; pound with a meat mallet to 1/8-in. thickness. Eliminate plastic wrap. Sprinkle with salt and pepper.

2. Spot five spinach leaves on every chicken bosom half. Spoon a meager 2 tablespoons of cream cheddar down the focal point of every chicken bosom half; sprinkle with 1 tablespoon pecans. Move up chicken; wrap up closes.
3. Unfurl puff baked good; cut into eight segments. Fold each into a 7-in. square. Spot chicken on one portion of each square; overlay other portion of baked good over chicken. Pleat edges with fork. Consolidate egg and cold water; brush over edges of cake.
4. Heat on a lubed 15x10x1-in. heating sheet until a thermometer peruses 165°, 20-25 minutes.

NUTRITION FACTS

- 1 serving: 624 calories, 32g fat (10g saturated fat), 136mg cholesterol, 742mg sodium, 39g carbohydrate (1g sugars, 6g fiber), 44g protein.

23. Sheet pan Lamb meal

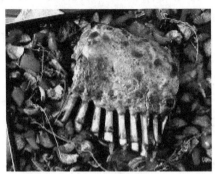

Prep Time 15 mins Cook Time 30 mins Total Time 45 mins

INGREDIENTS
- 2 ½ pounds lamb shoulder chops, see note below
- 1 large sweet potato
- 8 red new potatoes
- 2 Tablespoons olive oil
- 2 Tablespoons chopped fresh rosemary
- 1 Tablespoon chopped fresh thyme leaves
- Salt and freshly ground pepper
- 2 large garlic cloves, sliced
- 1 pint grape or cherry tomatoes
- 8 ounces frozen green peas

DIRECTION:
1. Preheat oven to 400ºF.
2. Trim the enormous bits of fat from the sheep and cut into 2-inch lumps.
3. Strip the yam and the new potatoes and cut into 2-inch lumps.
4. On an enormous rimmed sheet dish (12x17), throw the sheep and the potatoes with the olive oil, at that point sprinkle the spices over all and throw until equitably covered.

5. Add salt and pepper as you would prefer and throw. (At the point when I make this for my more distant family I leave it off by and large and let everybody add their own. My significant other loves salt and pepper, so when it's simply us, I use it liberally.)
6. Spread the meat and vegetables out on the plate equitably and dissipate the cut garlic on top.
7. Slide this into your preheated oven and meal for 20 minutes, throwing part of the way through cooking. Meat ought to be browned. (We like our sheep cooked medium-well. Assuming you need your meat more uncommon, start the potatoes and add the meat 5 to 10 minutes after the fact.)
8. Add the tomatoes and the peas to the sheet skillet and cook for an extra 10 minutes.
9. The store where I purchase my meat had 2 kinds of shoulder slashes, sharp edge and round bone. You need the hacks with the round bone, they are simpler to work with. Likewise, you can request that your butcher 3D shape the meat for you to save time at home.
10. In the event that you don't care for sheep, have a go at subbing sirloin steak. You may require less, in light of the fact that sirloin is less greasy than sheep.

NUTRITION FACTS
- 359 calories, 8g fat (4g saturated fat), 56mg cholesterol, 372mg sodium, 45g carbohydrate (19g sugars, 6g fiber), 31g protein. Diabetic Exchanges: 3 starch, 3 lean meat, 1 fat.

24. Roasted Halibut with Tahini Sauce

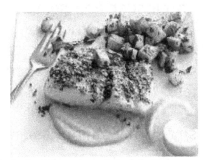

Total:40 mins Yield:Serves 4

INGREDIENTS
- 2 lemons
- 2 teaspoons zaatar*
- 1 teaspoon ground cumin
- 1 teaspoon red chile pieces
- 2 teaspoons genuine salt, partitioned
- ½ teaspoon pepper, separated
- 1 teaspoon extra-virgin olive oil
- 4 (1 in. thick) halibut filets (around 1/2 lbs.)
- ¼ cup tahini (sesame-seed paste)
- 1 garlic clove, stripped and crushed

DIRECTION
1. Stage 1
2. Set rack in top third of oven and preheat to 450°. Zing half of 1 lemon into a little bowl. Add zaatar, cumin, chile chips, 1 tsp. salt, 1/4 tsp. pepper, and the oil; blend. Coat one side of filets with paste.
3. Stage 2
4. Organize halibut, paste side up, on a heating sheet and set on upper rack. Broil until fish is simply cooked through, 6 to 10 minutes.

5. Stage 3
6. Put tahini, garlic, 2 tbsp. water, juice of 1/2 lemon, and remaining 1 tsp. salt and 1/4 tsp. pepper in a blender and spin until smooth and pourable. Add more lemon juice to taste, and more water on the off chance that you'd favor a more slender sauce. Cut remaining lemon into wedges.
7. Stage 4
8. Serve fish with tahini sauce and lemon wedges.
9. Stage 5
10. Find zaatar, a Middle Eastern zest mix of sesame seeds, sumac, thyme, and oregano, in your supermarket's flavor passageway.

NUTRITION FACTS

- Per Serving: 293 calories; calories from fat 44%; protein 38g; fat 14g; saturated fat 2.5g; carbohydrates 5.9g; fiber 1.7g; sodium 904mg; cholesterol 122mg.

25. Sheet pan Steak Bites

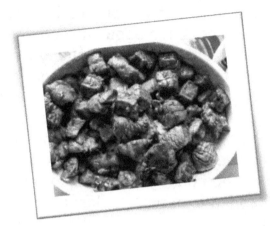

Prep Time: 10 mins Cook Time: 10 mins Total Time: 20 mins, 5 servings

INGREDIENTS
- 1 3/4 pounds flank steak
- 1/4 cup soy sauce
- 2 tablespoons nectar
- 1 tablespoon stew paste
- 1-2 tablespoons light seasoned olive oil

DIRECTION
1. Cut the steak across the grain into strips 1/2" wide. Cut each strip into reduced down pieces, roughly 1/2" – 3/4" in size. Spot the pieces of hamburger into a medium size bowl. Mix together the soy sauce, nectar, and bean stew paste. Pour over the meat and mix to cover well. Allow the meat to marinate for 20-30 minutes.
2. Heat a substantial base hardened steel dish or wok over medium high heat. At the point when

the dish is hot, add 1 tablespoon of oil and twirl to cover. Add 1/3 of the meat to the container and spread out in a solitary layer. Allow it to cook for about a moment, until the meat has carmelized. Flip the meat or throw with a spatula for an extra moment or two as it completes the process of cooking. Eliminate the meat from the dish to a plate.

3. Add half of the excess meat to the hot dish and rehash the above advances. Add the cooked meat to the holding up plate. In the event that vital, add the excess tablespoon of oil to the skillet prior to adding the leftover meat. Rehash the means. Enjoy!

4. In the event that anytime the skillet starts to smoke, it is excessively hot. Lower the heat marginally and keep cooking. Eliminate the steak chomps from the container when they are seared outwardly and still delicious within. They will keep cooking briefly after they are taken out from the heat. Skirt steak might be fill in for the flank steak in this formula.

NUTRITION FACTS

- Calories: 347kcal · Carbohydrates: 10g · Protein: 44g · Fat: 13g · Saturated Fat: 4g · Cholesterol: 119mg · Sodium: 916mg · Potassium: 722mg · Sugar: 9g · Vitamin C: 0.7mg · Calcium: 45mg · Iron: 3.4mg

26. Pan BEEF SALAD WITH ASIAN SLAW

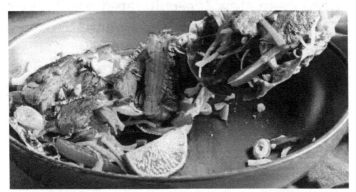

Prep Time:20 mins Cook Time:20 mins Total Time:40 mins Servings: 4 servings Calories: 384kcal

INGREDIENTS

- Marinated Beef
- 320 g sirloin steak (approx 2 steaks – fat eliminated)
- 2 tbsp clam sauce
- 1 tsp dim soy sauce
- 1 tbsp cornflour
- 1 tbsp sunflower oil
- Crunchy Slaw
- 400 g white cabbage (meagerly destroyed)
- 160 g mange promote (finely cut)
- 1 medium carrot (cut into fine cudgel)
- 1 red onion (finely cut)
- 1 red pepper (finely cut)
- Slaw Dressing
- 2 tbsp sunflower oil
- 1 tbsp light soy sauce
- 4 tbsp rice wine vinegar (can substitute with red wine vinegar)

- 2 tbsp lime juice
- 2 tsp sesame oil
- 1 clove garlic squashed
- 1 red bean stew (de-cultivated and finely cut)
- 1 tbsp root ginger (finely ground)
- 1 tbsp mint leaves (finely destroyed)
- To Serve
- 2 little jewel lettuce (forgets about isolated)
- 4 spring onions (finely cut)
- 4 tbsp peanuts (squashed)
- 1 lime (cut into wedges)
- 1 little bundle new mint leaves

DIRECTION

1. Marinated Beef
2. Spot the clam sauce, dim soy sauce and cornflour into a bowl and blend well to join to a smooth paste. Add the entire sirloin steaks to the marinade and blend to guarantee the steaks are totally covered. Put in a safe spot for 15 minutes while you set up the remainder of the dish.
3. Asian Slaw
4. Set up every one of the vegetables for the Asian slaw and spot them in an enormous bowl. Put in a safe spot.
5. In a bowl combine as one every one of the INGREDIENTS for the slaw dressing and mix well to join. Pour over the vegetables and blend completely through the vegetables. Put to the side until prepared to serve.
6. To serve
7. At the point when prepared to serve, place a huge non-stick griddle over a high heat. Add

1tbsp sunflower oil to the griddle and spot the steaks into the skillet to cook for 2-3 minutes on each side. The timeframe will change contingent upon the thickness of the steaks. However, for a medium cooked steak you are searching for an interior temperature of 60-65C.

8. At the point when the steak is cooked, eliminate from the container and put to the side on a warm plate to rest for 5 minutes.

9. In the interim set up the lettuce leaves and spot a spoon of the slaw into every one of the leaves.

10. When rested cut every sirloin steak into slender cuts and a few cuts onto every lettuce leaf. Trimming with spring onion, squashed peanuts, new torn mint leaves and a wedge of new lime. Serve right away.

11. On the off chance that you don't care for bean stew avoid it with regards to the dressing completely.

12. The trimming things are a serving idea in particular. In the event that you have a nut hypersensitivity leave the nuts off the dish.

NUTRITION FACTS

- Amount Per Serving
- Calories 384Calories from Fat 198
- % Daily Value*
- Fat 22g34%
- Saturated Fat 4g25%
- Cholesterol 49mg16%
- Sodium 667mg29%
- Potassium 880mg25%

- Carbohydrates 25g8%
- Fiber 7g29%
- Sugar 10g11%
- Protein 25g50%
- Vitamin A 5511IU110%
- Vitamin C 128mg155%
- Calcium 126mg13%
- Iron 4mg22%

27. Sheet pan Beef Lettuce Cups with Carrot & Daikon Slaw

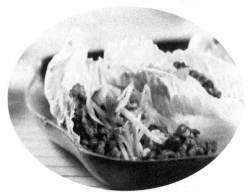

SERVINGS 4 PREP TIME 40 min COOK TIME 5 min DURATION 45 min

INGREDIENTS

- 1/4 cup rice vinegar
- 1 tbsp plus 1/2 tsp raw honey, divided
- 1/8 tsp sea salt
- 1 carrot, peeled and cut into matchsticks (1 cup)
- 1 daikon radish, cut into matchsticks (1 cup) (TIP: If you can't find daikon radish, regular radish works well here too.)
- 1 tsp sesame oil
- 10 oz lean ground beef
- 1/2 cup finely chopped red onion
- 3 cloves garlic, minced
- 1 tbsp peeled and minced fresh ginger
- 1 1/3 cups BPA-free canned unsalted black beans, drained and rinsed
- 1 tbsp reduced-sodium soy sauce
- 12 romaine lettuce leaves

- 2 tbsp chopped roasted unsalted peanuts
- 2 tbsp thinly sliced scallions

DIRECTION

1. Firstly In a medium bowl, whisk together vinegar, 1 tbsp honey and salt. Add carrot and radish; toss to coat. Cover and transfer to refrigerator to marinate until tender and chilled, at least 2 hours or overnight.
2. Heat a large nonstick skillet on medium and brush with oil. Then Add beef and sauté until no longer pink, about 5 minutes. Push beef to one side of skillet. To other side, add onion, garlic and ginger; sauté until onion softens, about 2 minutes.
3. Add beans, soy sauce and remaining 1/2 tsp honey and stir all INGREDIENTS together; simmer for 3 minutes, stirring occasionally.
4. Drain liquid from slaw. Fill in each lettuce leaf with 1/4 cup beef-bean mixture; top it with slaw. Garnish with peanuts and scallions.

NUTRITION FACTS

- Serving Size3 lettuce leaves, 3/4 cup beef mixture, 1/2 cup slaw
- Calories277
- Carbohydrate Content20 g
- Cholesterol Content46 mg
- Fat Content11 g
- Fiber Content7 g
- Protein Content21 g
- Saturated Fat Content3 g
- Sodium Content261 mg
- Sugar Content6 g
- Monounsaturated Fat Content0 g

- Polyunsaturated Fat Content0 g

28. Sheet Pan Seafood Bake with Buttery Wine Sauce

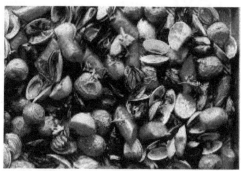

Active:15 mins Total:40 mins Yield:Serves 4 (serving size: about 5 1/3 oz.)

INGREDIENTS

- 12 ounces baby red potatoes
- 2 small yellow onions, cut into 1-in. wedges
- 2 lemons, halved crosswise
- 3 tablespoons olive oil
- 1 ½ teaspoons Cajun seafood boil seasoning (such as Slap Ya Mama Cajun Seafood Boil)
- 2 pounds littleneck clams in shells, scrubbed
- 12 ounces smoked andouille sausage, cut into 2-in. pieces
- 1 pound fresh mussels in shells, scrubbed
- ½ cup dry white wine
- ¼ cup salted butter, melted
- 1 tablespoon hot sauce (such as Crystal)
- 1 ½ teaspoons Worcestershire sauce
- 2 tablespoons chopped fresh flat-leaf parsley
- Lemon wedges, for serving

DIRECTION
1. Step 1

2. Preheat oven to 450°F with 1 rack in top third of oven and 1 rack in bottom third of oven. Toss together potatoes, onions, lemon halves, oil, and seafood boil seasoning on an aluminum-foil-lined rimmed baking sheet. Spread in an even layer, and roast in preheated oven on bottom rack until potatoes are just tender, about 25 minutes.
3. Step 2
4. Spread clams on a second foil-lined rimmed baking sheet. Bake at 450°F on top rack just until clams begin to open, 8 to 10 minutes.
5. Step 3
6. When potatoes have roasted 25 minutes and clams have opened, spread andouille evenly on baking sheet with potatoes, and spread mussels evenly over clams. Pour wine over clam mixture. Bake until mussels have opened, about 8 minutes.
7. Step 4
8. Stir together butter, hot sauce, and Worcestershire sauce. Spread potato mixture evenly over clams and mussels on baking sheet. Drizzle evenly with butter sauce, and sprinkle evenly with parsley. Garnish with lemon wedges, and serve immediately.

NUTRITION FACTS
- Per serving (6 servings)
- Calories:347
- Fat:19 g
- Saturated fat:6 g
- Carbohydrates:11 g
- Sugar:6 g

- Fiber:1 g
- Protein:32 g
- Sodium:979 mg
- Cholesterol:99 mg

29. Baked Lobster Tails with Citrus-Herb Butter

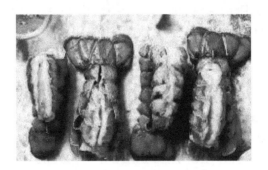

Active:20 mins Total:20 mins Yield:Serves 4 (serving size: 1 lobster tail)

INGREDIENTS

- 4 (5 oz.) new lobster tails
- ½ cup (4 oz.) unsalted spread, dissolved and isolated
- 2 teaspoons new lemon juice (from 1 lemon)
- 1 teaspoon finely chopped new tarragon
- 1 teaspoon finely chopped new level leaf parsley
- 1 teaspoon daintily cut new chives
- ½ teaspoon finely chopped garlic (from 1 garlic clove)
- ¼ teaspoon legitimate salt
- Lemon wedges, for serving

DIRECTION

1. Stage 1
2. Preheat oven to 450°F. Using kitchen shears, cut straight down top focus of lobster tail shell. Utilize a spoon to delicately deliver lobster meat from each side of shell. Delicately pull

meat away from lower part of lobster, and spot on top of shells. Spot lobster tails on a preparing sheet fixed with material paper, and spoon 1 tablespoon of the margarine over each. Prepare in preheated oven until dazzling red and dark, 12 to 14 minutes.

3. Stage 2
4. In the interim, heat remaining 1/4 cup dissolved margarine in a little pot over medium-low. At the point when prepared to serve, eliminate spread from heat, and move to a little serving bowl. Mix in lemon juice, tarragon, parsley, chives, garlic, and salt. Serve lobster tails with citrus-spice margarine and lemon wedges.

NUTRITION FACTS
• Calories: 1077 kcal Carbohydrates: 91 g Protein: 57 g Fat: 51 g Saturated fat: 28 g Sodium: 1057 mg Potassium: 1204 mg Fiber: 5 g Sugar: 5 g Vitamin A: 2600 IE Vitamin C: 89.2 mg Calcium : 119 mg Iron: 3.5

30. Sheet pan Hoisin Beef

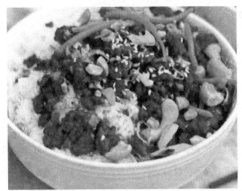

Servings: 4 to 6 Prep Time: 20 Minutes Cook Time: 10 Minutes Total Time: 30 Minutes

INGREDIENTS

- 2 pounds 90% lean ground meat
- 3/4 teaspoon preparing pop
- 6 tablespoons hoisin sauce, best quality like Lee Kum Kee or Kikkoman (use sans gluten if necessary)
- 3 tablespoons soy sauce (use without gluten if necessary)
- 1 tablespoon tomato paste
- 1 teaspoon Asian sesame oil
- 1 teaspoon sugar
- 1/2 teaspoon red pepper pieces
- 1 tablespoon vegetable oil
- 4 cloves garlic, chopped
- 2 tablespoons chopped new ginger
- 5 scallions, cut, light and dull green parts isolated
- FOR SERVING
- Rice
- Chopped cashews

- Sesame seeds
- Destroyed veggies, like carrots, lettuce or chime peppers

DIRECTION

1. In a pan, using your hands, squash the meat with the preparing pop. Allow it to sit on the counter for 20-25 minutes.
2. In the interim, in a little bowl, mix together the hoisin sauce, soy sauce, tomato paste, sesame oil, sugar, and red pepper pieces. Put in a safe spot.
3. When the meat is "dealt with" and prepared to cook, heat the vegetable oil in a huge sauté dish over medium-high heat. Earthy colored the meat, mixing as often as possible and breaking into pieces, until just somewhat pink, around 5 minutes. (I don't deplete the fat - there's not so much and it adds flavor.)
4. Add the garlic, ginger, and light scallions. Cook, blending habitually, until mollified, a couple of moments.
5. Add the held hoisin sauce blend and cook until the meat is all around covered and cooked through, about a moment. Taste and change preparing if essential.
6. Tenderly mix in the leftover scallions and spoon the hamburger into astonishes rice. Top with sesame seeds, chopped cashews, and destroyed veggies, in the event that you like.
7. Note: To complete this dish shortly, hack the garlic, ginger, and scallions while the meat is being treated with heating pop.

8. Cooler Friendly DIRECTION The meat blend can be frozen for as long as 3 months. Reheat in the microwave or on the burner.

NUTRITION FACTS
- Per serving (6 servings)
- Calories:347
- Fat:19 g
- Saturated fat:6 g
- Carbohydrates:11 g
- Sugar:6 g
- Fiber:1 g
- Protein:32 g
- Sodium:979 mg
- Cholesterol:99 mg

31. Sheet Pan Thai Red Curry Mussels

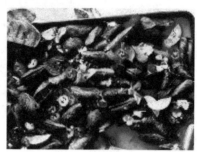

Active:10 mins Total:20 mins Yield:Serves 4

INGREDIENTS

- 2 pounds mussels, scoured and debearded
- 1 (14-oz.) would coconut be able to drain
- ½ cup dry white wine
- 1 (4-oz.) container red curry paste
- 1 teaspoon garlic paste
- 1 teaspoon ginger paste
- 1 teaspoon lemongrass paste
- 1 tablespoon chopped new cilantro
- 1 tablespoon chopped new level leaf parsley
- Flame broiled crusty bread cuts
- Trimmings: lime wedges, cilantro twigs, Thai basil springs, red Fresno chile cuts, and jalapeño chile cuts

DIRECTION

1. Stage 1
2. Preheat oven to 400°F. Pick over mussels, disposing of any that are broken. Spot all remaining mussels on a rimmed sheet skillet.
3. Stage 2

4. Whisk together coconut milk, wine, curry paste, garlic paste, ginger paste, and lemongrass paste in a medium bowl until smooth. Pour equally over mussels.
5. Stage 3
6. Prepare in preheated oven until every one of the mussels have opened, around 10 minutes. Sprinkle with cilantro and parsley. Present with barbecued bread; top with wanted toppings.

NUTRITION FACTS

- Calories: 287cal (14%)Carbohydrates: 21g (7%)Protein: 27g (54%)Fat: 11g (17%)Saturated Fat: 1g (6%)Trans Fat: 1gCholesterol: 80mg (27%)Sodium: 948mg (41%)Potassium: 522mg (15%)Fiber: 1g (4%)Sugar: 18g (20%)Vitamin A: 59IU (1%)Vitamin C: 13mg (16%)Calcium: 15mg (2%)Iron: 1mg (6%)

32. Pan Chicken Tequila

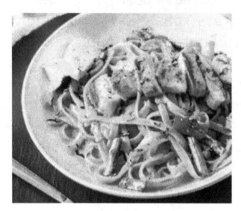

INGREDIENTS
- 1-2 pounds dry spinach fettuccine (or 2 pounds fresh)
- 1/2 cup chopped cilantro (2 tablespoons for garnish/finishing)
- 2-tablespoons of chopped fresh garlic
- 2-tablespoons chopped jalapeno pepper (seeds and veins can be removed if a milder flavor is desired)
- 3-tablespoons unsalted butter (reserve tablespoons per container)
- 1/2 cup of chicken stock
- 2-tablespoons of tequila
- 2-tablespoons of freshly squeezed lime juice
- 3-tablespoons of soy sauce
- 1/2 pound chicken breast diced 3/4 inch
- 1/4 cup red onion thinly sliced
- 1 1/2 cup of red bell pepper thinly sliced
- 1/2 cup of yellow bell pepper thinly sliced
- 1/2 cup green pepper thinly sliced
- 1 1/2 cups of cream

DIRECTION

1. Quickly prepare to boil salted water for cooking pasta; cook dinner al dente, for dry pasta for 8 to 10 minutes, for bubbly for about three minutes. Pasta can be cooked, rinsed, and oiled slightly ahead of time, after which it is "flashed" in boiling water or cooked to match the sauce/topping.

2. Mix 1/3 cup of cilantro, garlic, and jalapeno over medium heat in 2 tablespoons of oil for four to 5 minutes. Remove lime juice, tequila, and stock. Bring the combination to a boil and cook to a pasty consistency until reduced; put aside.

3. Pour over the diced soy sauce; Set aside for 5 minutes. Meanwhile, prepare evening onions and peppers with the last of butter over medium heat, stirring occasionally. Toss and add the reserved vegetables and cream when the vegetable wilt (go limp), add the chook and soy sauce.

4. Bring the sauce to a boil; cook gently until the chicken has melted and the sauce is thick (about 3 minutes).

NUTRITION FACTS

- Calories: 1077 kcal Carbohydrates: 91 g Protein: 57 g Fat: 51 g Saturated fat: 28 g Sodium: 1057 mg Potassium: 1204 mg Fiber: 5 g Sugar: 5 g Vitamin A: 2600 IE Vitamin C: 89.2 mg Calcium : 119 mg Iron: 3.5

33. Fish Tacos with Lime-Cilantro Cremal

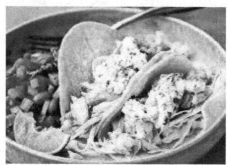

Total:15 mins Yield:4 servings (serving size: 2 tacos)
INGREDIENTS

- Crema:
- ¼ cup daintily cut green onions
- ¼ cup chopped new cilantro
- 3 tablespoons without fat mayonnaise
- 3 tablespoons decreased fat sharp cream
- 1 teaspoon ground lime skin
- 1 ½ teaspoons new lime juice
- ¼ teaspoon salt
- 1 garlic clove, minced
- Tacos:
- 1 teaspoon ground cumin
- 1 teaspoon ground coriander
- ½ teaspoon smoked paprika
- ¼ teaspoon ground red pepper
- ⅛ teaspoon salt
- ⅛ teaspoon garlic powder
- 1 ½ pounds red snapper filets
- Cooking shower
- 8 (6-inch) corn tortillas
- 2 cups shredded cabbage

DIRECTION
1. Stage 1
2. Preheat oven to 425°.
3. Stage 2
4. To plan crema, consolidate the initial 8 INGREDIENTS in a little bowl; put in a safe spot.
5. Stage 3
6. To get ready tacos, consolidate cumin and next 5 INGREDIENTS (through garlic powder) in a little bowl; sprinkle zest combination uniformly over the two sides of fish. Spot fish on a heating sheet covered with cooking shower. Prepare at 425° for 9 minutes or until fish chips effectively when tried with a fork or until wanted level of doneness. Spot fish in a bowl; break into pieces with a fork. Heat tortillas as per bundle DIRECTION. Separation fish uniformly among tortillas; top each with 1/4 cup cabbage and 1 tablespoon cremal.

NUTRITION FACTS
- Per Serving: 394 calories; calories from fat 14%; fat 6.3g; saturated fat 1.5g; mono fat 1.5g; poly fat 1.5g; protein 40.3g; carbohydrates 40.1g; fiber 5.5g; cholesterol 70mg; iron 3.5mg; sodium 857mg; calcium 233mg.

34. Honey-Mustard Baked Salmon with Vegetables

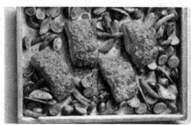

Active:15 mins Total:30 mins Yield:Serves 4

INGREDIENTS
- 1 pound child red potatoes, split (3 cups)
- 3 shallots, quartered longwise (around 1 cup)
- 4 tablespoons olive oil, partitioned
- 1 teaspoon genuine salt, partitioned
- 3 tablespoons in addition to 2 tsp. entire grain mustard, partitioned
- 1 ½ teaspoons nectar, partitioned
- ½ cup panko breadcrumbs
- 2 teaspoons chopped new thyme
- 4 (5-oz.) skin-on salmon filets
- 3 cups new sugar snap peas, managed
- 2 teaspoons red wine vinegar
- 1 teaspoon ground garlic
- ¼ teaspoon smoked paprika

DIRECTION
1. Stage 1
2. Preheat oven to 425°F. Throw together potatoes, shallots, 1 tablespoon of the oil, and 1⊠ teaspoon of the salt on a huge rimmed preparing sheet. Organize combination in an even layer, with potatoes confronting cut sides

down. Cook until practically delicate, around 15 minutes. Eliminate from oven.
3. Stage 2
4. While potato blend broils, mix together 3 tablespoons of the mustard, 1/4 teaspoon of the salt, and 1 teaspoon of the nectar in a little bowl. Mix together panko, thyme, 1 tablespoon of the oil, and 1/4 teaspoon of the salt in a different little bowl. Mastermind salmon filets, skin side down, on a plate. Spread mustard combination equally over skinless highest points of filets. Sprinkle best equally with panko combination, squeezing to follow.
5. Stage 3
6. Mix cooked potato combination on heating sheet, pushing blend toward edges of preparing sheet with a spatula. Spot salmon filets, skin side down, in focus of preparing sheet. Spread sugar snap peas equally around salmon. Return preparing sheet to oven. Heat at 425°F until panko outside is brilliant brown, salmon is cooked to medium doneness (turns flaky and misty), and potatoes are delicate, around 10 minutes.
7. Stage 4
8. In the interim, whisk together vinegar, garlic, smoked paprika, and remaining 2 tablespoons oil, 1/4 teaspoon salt, 2 teaspoons mustard, and 1/2 teaspoon nectar in a little bowl until consolidated.
9. Stage 5
10. Separate salmon filets and vegetable combination equally among 4 plates. Sprinkle vegetable blend equally with vinaigrette.

NUTRITION FACTS

- 1 serving: 400 calories, 23g fat (4g saturated fat), 85mg cholesterol, 535mg sodium, 13g carbohydrate (3g sugars, 3g fiber), 32g protein. Diabetic Exchanges: salmon , 1-1/2 fat, 1 vegetable.

CONCLUSION

Hope you all enjoyed delicious sheet pan recipes. Making your own dinner is much more grounded than eating out or mentioning takeaway. You will use less salt, and less sad fats, while adding colossal heaps of brilliant veggies to your protein in these recipes. Try at home and appreciate. God luck!

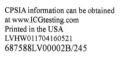